101 REASONS TO SMILE

DR. HOWARD B. SHULLMAN, DMD

StarGroup Books, West Palm Beach, Florida

Concept and supervision: Brenda Star

Book design and graphic art: Mel Abfier

Editor: Chris Seal

Proofreader: Tracy Carvalho

Published by StarGroup International, Inc.
561.547.0667
www.stargroupinternational.com

Printed in Canada

Library of Congress Cataloging-in-Publication 2017958665

101 Reasons to Smile
ISBN 978-1-884886-43-0

TABLE OF CONTENTS

ACKNOWLEDGEMENTS

To my patients: I would like to express my deepest gratitude to the thousands of committed patients who continue to support my orthodontic practice with so much enthusiasm and excitement. I thank you for your trust and confidence; allowing me to perform dentistry for you is a privilege. I take my responsibility and my patient relationship seriously, and my goal is always to deliver to you the SMILE of your dreams.

To my amazing team at Shullman Orthodontics: It is my privilege to share this amazing journey together. Your belief in my vision and your energy to treat our patients with the utmost quality and customer service, is inspiring. I offer a special thanks to my marketing coordinator, Chris Seal, who wouldn't let me off the hook and encouraged me to fulfill my commitment to complete this project.

To my book production team: I give a special thanks to Brenda Star and Mel Abfier of StarGroup International for their creative direction in producing this book. They are true professionals whose work ethic and personal concern made it happen.

To my children, Maddie, Emma, and Kate: You are all extraordinary. You have given me more than you have received in ways only a father can truly know. You are the reason I push so hard each and every day to do what I do, and I'm proud to watch you grow into beautiful ladies.

To my best friend and dear wife, Deanna: Thank you from the bottom of my heart for your unconditional loving support. I admire you and appreciate your beauty, grace, and love. You have allowed me to put much of my time and energy into growing my orthodontic practice while you work so hard to keep our three beautiful girls moving through life. I cannot thank you enough.

INTRODUCTION

Smiles inspire all of us. Smiles evoke confidence. Smiles warm the soul. Smiles have the ability to change our mood and the mood of others. Smiles are contagious. For these reasons and so many more, this book was written to express the joy I have experienced over the years creating beautiful smiles that last a lifetime.

HEARING YOUR CHILD SAY, "MOMMY" FOR THE FIRST TIME.

Getting a **letter** in the mail from your child while they're at sleep-away **camp**.

Coming home from a long day at work to see

your dog wagging his tail in anticipation.

BEING ABLE TO BUTTON UP THOSE JEANS

Seeing your children snuggle with each other.

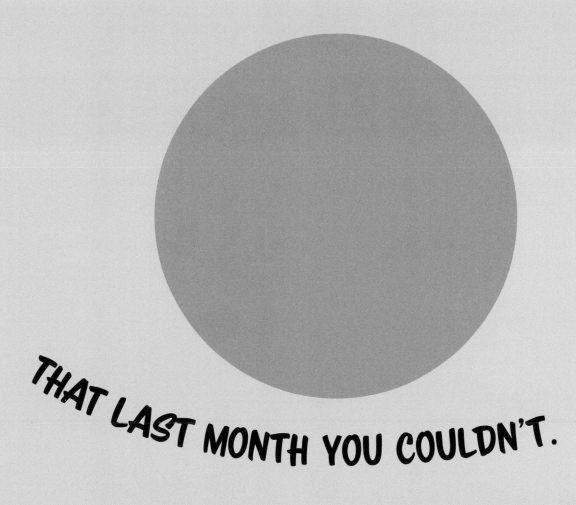

THAT LAST MONTH YOU COULDN'T.

Listening to a story being told by someone

Seeing that same couple holding

who has been in love for 50 years.

hands as they tell their story.

catching that first fish with your grandpa.

Watching your child make their first free throw.

Kicking off that second ski on your favorite lake and

Driving down a
back country road
listening to your
favorite acoustic
playlist.

sliding your foot behind the other.

Smelling the orange blossoms in the air as you

cruise down the road on your motorcycle.

Walking into a room where all your family and

friends jump out and scream,

SURPRISE!!

TAKING **BRACES** OFF A CHILD WHO HAD NO

WITNESSING THAT SAME CHILD SEE THEIR

DESIRE TO SMILE AND FACE THE WORLD.

DREAMS BECOME A REALITY WITH A BRAND NEW SMILE.

Smelling that first pot of coffee brewing

Allowing your child to "help" you load the dishwasher when you know you'll have to redo it once they leave the room.

on a cool autumn morning.

BOWLING YOUR FIRST STRIKE!

KNOWING THAT SOMEONE TRULY LOVES YOU.

Seeing
your
child
ride a
bike
for
the
first
time.

**Squishing your toes
in the sand
as the ocean water
surrounds your feet.**

Hearing the words, "I Love You" for the first time.

Stepping into a hot bath to feel the stresses of the day melt away.

Getting that first paycheck.

Glancing in the

mirror to see that you're having a good hair day.

Sacrificing your seat for someone who

needs it more than you.

Going out on your first date.

Waking up to realize
you have **nothing** to do
that **day**.

Looking into someone's eyes and seeing their soul.

Hearing the words, "It's a girl".

Waking up to your dog

Hearing your child say,
"Daddy" for the first time.

licking your toes.

Hugs from your kids after being

away several days for work.

Watching your child walk down the aisle with their high school sweetheart.

Giving yourself a challenge and exceeding your goal.

KNOWING YOUR KIDS ARE IN GOOD HANDS WITH GRANDMA AS YOU HEAD OUT FOR THE WEEKEND.

Watching your favorite football team win the game on a last second Hail Mary.

Making memories with your grandparents.

Watching your child's face as they

see straight A's on their report card.

A HOT SHOWER TO BEGIN A NEW DAY.

Listening to your child sing their favorite song.

53

Because you've had a heck of
a week and it's Friday!

It's summer **vacation** and you're heading out on

a 10 day **road** trip with the family.

Hearing a joke told by your child.

Wrapping yourself up in a blanket fresh out of the dryer.

Being picked up at the airport by someone you haven't seen in a long time.

Racing down the mountain on snow

ski's achieving your best time ever.

Giving back to your community.

Looking through

old family photos or videos.

Your dentist telling you that you are cavity-free.

Watching your wife give birth to your first child.

Finding money in your pocket that you forgot was there.

Getting approved for your first home mortgage.

Getting in your bed after a long exhausting day.

Giving a complete stranger a hug.

Driving your first car.

Fresh baked
chocolate chip
cookies.

Delivering Flowers To Someone Who Needs Support, But Would Never Ask For It.

Making the final payment on your loan and having no more debt.

Seeing your daughter perform

Waking up to find your kids jumping in bed with

her first **dance** solo.

you and snuggling under the covers.

Passing a yearly health physical with flying colors.

Witnessing a shooting star dance across the midnight sky.

Watching your child tie their shoes for the first time.

Seeing your
first born child
in the arms of
their mother.

Feeling the
warmth of
the sun as
it shines on
your cold
face.

Watching your baby take their first step.

Watching your child
score a goal on the
soccer field.

Listening to your favorite 80's rock ballad.

UNLOCKING THE DOOR TO YOUR BRAND NEW HOUSE.

Unwrapping an
unexpected gift from
a new friend.

WITNESSING A RANDOM ACT OF KINDNESS.

Checking off
the last item
on your bucket
list!

Opening the door for someone.

Receiving a text
from an
old friend.

The sound of rain falling on a tin roof

Walking up to the stage and receiving your diploma.

Cutting open a *pumpkin* to reveal the soon-to-be **roasted** pumpkin seeds.

It's 6 a.m. and you're **done** with your **workout** for the day.

Road trips with the family.

KNOWING THAT TOMORROW IS GOING TO BE A NEW DAY.

Seeing your first snowflake falling from a winter sky.

Receiving a call from your best friend when you needed to hear their voice so badly.

Reaching out with your *hand*

Zero balance on your credit card...

to lift someone up.

is that even possible?

A night with no homework.

Living a life with purpose.

Walking into that
job interview
fully prepared.

Seeing the work you do impact people in a positive, lasting way.

RUNNING INTO A FRIEND YOU HAVEN'T SEEN IN YEARS.

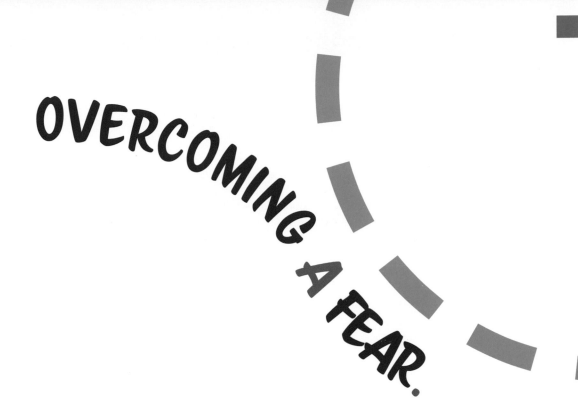

OVERCOMING A FEAR.

Sharing a warm meal with someone in need.

Seeing someone get engaged.

Hearing that your child aced their standardized testing.

The feeling of accomplishment after you go to the gym.

Holding someone's hand for the first time.

Someone holding the door for you.

Catching a glimpse of yourself dancing in the mirror.

Tasting something delicious for the first time.

Seeing an "A" on that math test you were dreading.

Watching as your child figures out a problem all on their own.

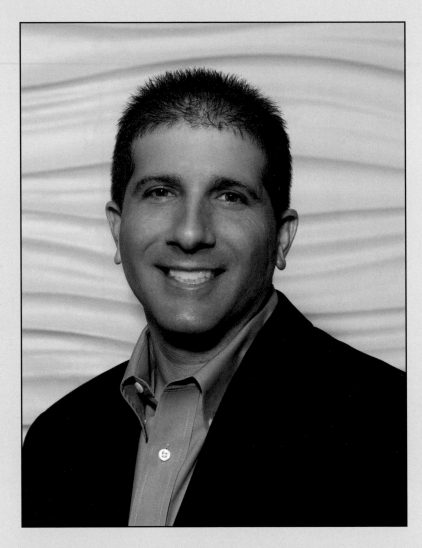

As a doctor, I treat patients whose ages, situations and needs vary, but I recognize that each one has placed a great deal of trust in me and my team. I value each and every patient relationship.

About Dr. Howard B. Shullman

Born and raised in Miami, Florida, Dr. Shullman attended the University of Florida where he received his undergraduate degree in bio-medical engineering. Eager for more Gator football, he stayed in Gainesville to earn his Doctorate of Dental Medicine degree.

Following graduation, he practiced general dentistry in Tampa, Florida, focusing on the treatment of children, before continuing his orthodontic training at Nova Southeastern University. There he served as Chief Resident in the Department of Orthodontics during his final year.

His love of the constantly evolving field of orthodontics drives him to be knowledgeable about the newest treatments. His patients can get the most up-to-date and effective care. Dr. Shullman is active in the Wellington community where he supports and contributes to the local schools and recreational leagues. He is frequently invited to speak in classrooms to educate children about basic hygiene.

He offers internships to high school and college students interested in the dental field, and provides office tours for area Girl Scout troops.

Dr. Shullman married his wife, Deanna, in December, 2000. They have three beautiful daughters – Maddie, Emma, and Kate. The family enjoys an active lifestyle that includes golfing, boating, hiking, skiing, and traveling.

ABOUT THE PRACTICE

PHILOSOPHY OF CARE

Our top priority is to provide you with the highest quality orthodontic care in a friendly, comfortable environment. With over 100 years combined experience, the staff at Shullman Orthodontics is more than qualified to ensure that you receive the best orthodontic care available.

We are passionate about orthodontics and dedicated to working one-on-one with you and your family to build a strong, lasting relationship. Whether you're an adult, adolescent, or child, we are committed to helping you achieve the smile you deserve – a healthy, beautiful one!

No two smiles are alike. We recognize that each patient has different needs that can only be met with a unique treatment plan. We pride ourselves in offering courteous service to everyone who walks through our doors. As a new patient, you will receive a complimentary "Dr. Shullman Smile Assessment." This is a comprehensive look at the health of your teeth as we evaluate your smile goals. This important initial visit includes an office tour, a complete exam with x-rays, and a treatment consultation with Dr. Shullman. Your smile assessment provides a complete clinical diagnosis and a detailed treatment plan, including cost estimates.

Because we want you, our patients, to look your best and feel confident about your smile, we offer a variety of orthodontic solutions customized to fit your needs. Options include clear or metal braces, SureSmile, Invisalign, and Invisalign Teen.

EXTENSIVE EXPERIENCE & KNOWLEDGE

Since 2005, Dr. Shullman has transformed over 5,000 smiles and helped to instill self-confidence in people throughout Palm Beach County. With his commitment to changing lives, he brings excellence and compassion to all of his patients every day.

Dr. Shullman's excellent education, experience, and dedication earn him constant referrals from patients and also from other dentists and doctors.

To ensure that he always provides cutting-edge treatments in the ever-changing field of orthodontics, he spends over 150 hours yearly in continuing education coursework. The office staff attends classes on a quarterly basis, taught by industry leaders.

ADVANCED TECHNOLOGY

Shullman Orthodontics provides the latest orthodontic technology to ensure top-quality care for every patient, which includes providing the most advanced orthodontic diagnostic and treatment technology, such as:

• iTero Digital Impression System — No More Gagging — Thanks to the revolutionary iTero scanning technology, you no longer have to bite down or gag on uncomfortable molds to get an impression of your teeth. The iTero's scanner uses laser technology to capture a highly accurate 3D image of the individual characteristics of your teeth and gum tissues. The completed scan converts to a 3D model that helps Dr. Shullman design the most precise, efficient treatment plan for your teeth.

• iCAT Dental Imaging—Shullman Orthodontics is our area's very first orthodontic practice to use the state-of-the-art iCAT cone beam 3-D dental imaging system to obtain high definition, 3D images of the mouth, face, and jaw. The iCAT technology replaces the traditional two-dimensional x-rays normally taken, allowing more accurate identification and diagnosis of any issues affecting orthodontic treatment.

WE RESPECT YOUR TIME

Your time is valuable. That's why we do our utmost to respect your time when you come to see us. Here are a few ways that we strive to provide you with a streamlined experience at our office:

• No Wait Times – When you visit our office you can count on being seen on time. We understand that you don't have hours to wait for your appointment, so we've created an environment in which appointments run smoothly and efficiently each day.

• Late Evening & Weekend Appointments – With work, school, and other activities, we know it can be tough for you to make an appointment during regular daytime hours. That's why we offer extended times and weekend appointments for your convenience.

• Same Day Appointments – Some orthodontic offices may not have availability for days, if not weeks! At Shullman Orthodontics, we maintain an organized and efficient schedule, so we can offer you an appointment on the same day that you call us.

• Same Day Treatment Starts – Some orthodontists only provide diagnosis during the initial consultation, requiring a patient to schedule a new appointment to actually start orthodontic treatment. We think that is a waste of your time and money! That's why we will begin your treatment on the same day as your "Dr. Shullman Smile Assessment."

SPANISH-SPEAKING CARE

Committed to offering quality care to every person in the Wellington area who needs it, we provide our services to the Spanish-speaking community.

CARING FOR OUR COMMUNITY

We are grateful for the opportunity to serve patients like you! It is important to Dr. Shullman that he gives back to you and our local community.

In addition, Shullman Orthodontics is proud to announce the launch of a new community outreach program, Smiles Matter, emBrace it! We will partner with several charitable agencies and local schools who will identify and screen families that are unable to afford needed orthodontic care. Our goal is to donate $1,000,000 in orthodontic services – that's a lot of smiles for kids in Palm Beach County!

MADE IN THE USA

We take great pride in the services we provide to the Palm Beach County area. That's why we only use quality braces that are made to the highest clinical manufacturing standards, right here in America.

When you choose us for your orthodontic treatment, you can have confidence that the materials used will provide lasting results.

PATIENT REWARDS

Shullman Orthodontics is devoted not only to offering exceptional service and results, but also to making treatment fun and rewarding. Through contests and individual treatment goal challenges, our Patient Rewards Card Program encourages our patients to reach – and exceed – their treatment goals. The prizes we award create a great deal of excitement!

Call us or visit our website to find out about our latest programs and prizes! This is just another way that we focus on making your treatment a positive, rewarding experience.

MULTIPLE GUARANTEES

Lifetime Satisfaction Guarantee – Shullman Orthodontics offers exceptional orthodontic treatment and we are confident that you will love your new smile — in fact, we guarantee it! If you are unhappy with your results at any point after your orthodontic treatment, simply let us know, and we will fix it.

Lifetime Retainer Guarantee – The key to lasting treatment results is properly wearing and maintaining your orthodontic retainer. Most orthodontists will charge a fee to replace a retainer, but we know that sometimes accidents happen. If you lose or break your retainer, Dr. Shullman will replace it for FREE.

AFFORDABLE PAYMENT OPTIONS

When it comes to our braces or our payment plans, we don't have a "one size fits all" policy. Dr. Shullman never wants a patient to resort to sub-par treatment due to financial concerns. That's why we offer finance options that will fit every budget and give you something to smile about! If you don't have orthodontic insurance, we currently partner with OrthoFi to offer flexible payment plans.

TESTIMONIALS

Absolutely EVERYTHING is done with an excellence and attention to detail that you just cannot find elsewhere! Not only were Dr. Shullman and his staff attentive to what I hoped to achieve from my Invisalign journey, but they truly were sincere in helping me achieve the best smile possible. Friendly doctor and staff who always keep their patients in mind. Would definitely recommend to everyone reading this!!

Kaddie M.

Dr. Shullman felt it was too soon to begin treatment. We were instructed to wait. How refreshing to have an honest assessment!

Nathan R.

My son loves seeing Dr. Shullman and his staff! He was apprehensive about going to the orthodontist at first, but now that he has gotten to know them, he feels very comfortable there. He's doing so well with treatment that he's months ahead of schedule!

Shawn T.

The Staff and Dr. Shullman are always so accommodating and helpful, especially after hours .

Stacy V.

I always have a pleasant experience with Dr. Shullman. He took good care of my older daughter with braces and now regularly checks my younger daughter to determine the best time to start her treatment. He is never rushed, always takes time to explain the process and the staff is awesome with the kids. I would highly recommend him to all my friends and family.

Jeff Y.

My child got very emotional when she saw her braces for the first time. I do not think she expected to feel that way. Suzie (orthodontic assistant) was very supportive and kind. She was very caring and attentive to my sensitive 12 year old.

Jolie I.

I am so happy that we shopped around and found this office. It is night and day compared to any of the other 4 we visited!

Michael H.

When Taylor's braces were coming off we were both sad because Dr. Shullman and his staff are excellent and made us feel like family. When we knew that we had 1 year with the retainers we were alright. I will refer anyone I know who are looking for a good orthodontist.

DaNette & Taylor D.

I like the modern technology, the bottled water, and not having to wait for my appointments... I like everything! You guys are great!

Laurie C.

The office runs very smoothly and efficiently; a clean and aesthetic environment. I appreciate the up-to-date technology, the website, email reminders and the Google calendar.

Elaynah E.

Shullman Orthodontist is a place where they welcome me with joy. I've had my braces now for over a year and they have made my smile even bigger and better. My experience at Shullman's is great. Everyone that knows me knows I like to smile so when my braces are off look out world because there is no stopping this smiling child!

Jasmine Y.

We recently finished up my daughter's two year treatment and we couldn't be more pleased. Not only do her teeth look beautiful but Shullman Orthodontics made the entire experience a pleasure. Their office is beyond organized and the staff helpful and friendly. We actually look forward to starting our younger daughter very soon!!

Kris R.

The staff is amazing! Dr. Shullman is the best! He is very generous and genuine. This office has made my child not hate going to the orthodontist! Thank you!

Meroe R.

Dr. Shullman's practice has the friendliest, most professional staff. They are always smiling and accommodating to their little patients! My son is always excited when he knows he has an appointment with Dr. Shullman, and we are thankful to have such an exceptional orthodontist in our area! I wouldn't refer my friends to anyone else!

Rema A.

I like the warm and professional environment, personable staff, and never a wait. You make the whole process from consultation a truly pleasant one.

Eve G.

The entire experience at Shullman Orthodontics is highly professional. Dr. Shullman and staff take the time to ensure the kids aren't pushed into treatment and work to minimize time in treatment with the best possible outcome. I have two children in their care and am extremely satisfied!

Michelle T.